DIABETIC COOKBOOKS FOR TYPE 2 DIABETES

Flavorful Recipes to Manage Your Blood Sugar

T. John

COPYRIGHT PAGE

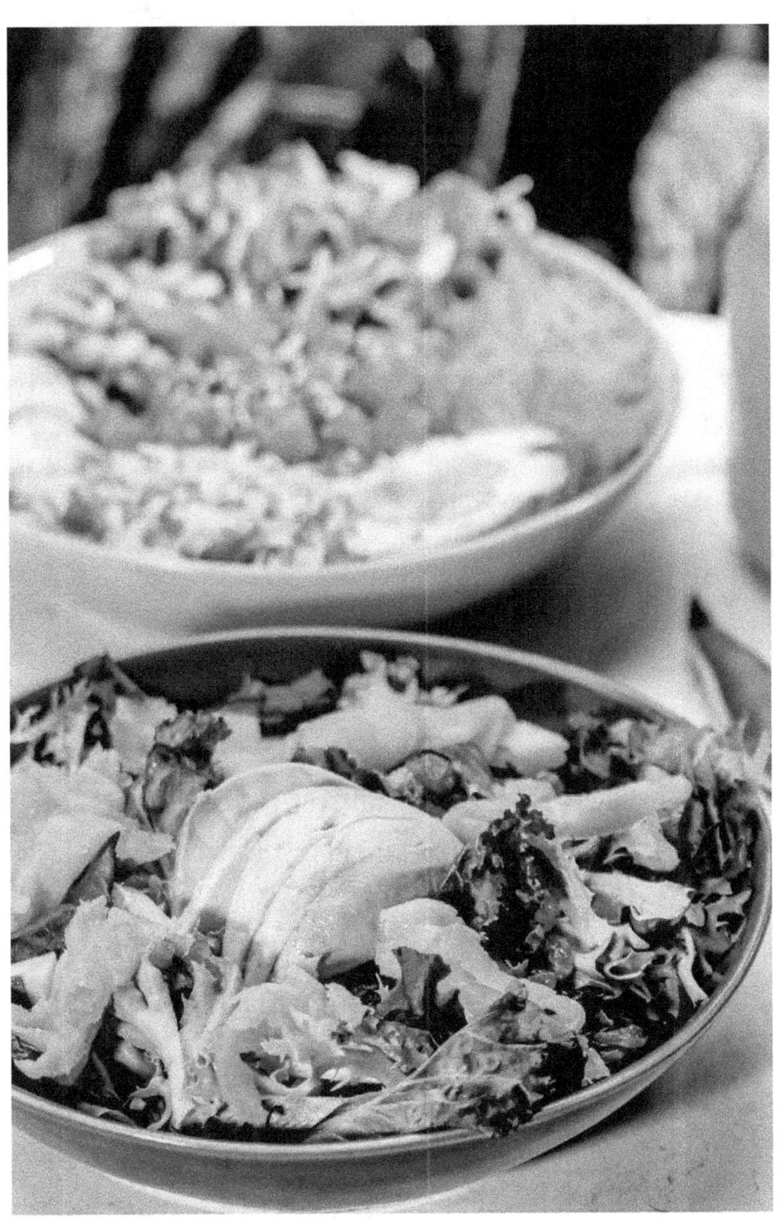

TABLE OF CONTENTS

Chapter 5: Snacks and Appetizers 84

CONCLUSION 135

INTRODUCTION

Imagine your body as a bustling city, with glucose as the fuel powering every corner. In type 2 diabetes, the traffic jam comes early – your body struggles to use glucose efficiently, causing havoc on the streets. But unlike an urban gridlock, this isn't an unsolvable mess. Enter the hero: nutrition.

Understanding the Diabetes-Diet Dance:

First, let's break down the villain: carbohydrates. Carbs act like fast-food restaurants – quick bursts of energy that leave you wanting more. In diabetes, these spikes in blood sugar are the troublesome traffic jams. But carbs aren't the enemy! Choose whole grains, veggies, and legumes - think artisanal bakeries and organic farmers' markets - slow-burning, nutrient-rich fuel that keeps your city humming smoothly.

Tips for Blood Sugar Smooth Sailing:

- **Portion Patrol**: Picture your plate as a dial. Fill half with non-starchy veggies (the leafy greens and colorful bell peppers), a quarter with protein (grilled chicken or lentil stew), and the remaining quarter with whole grains (brown rice or quinoa).This balanced composition keeps your blood sugar singing like a well-rehearsed orchestra.

- **Fiber First**: Think of fiber as the traffic cops, directing sugar into your system at a steady pace. Load up on those veggies, fruits, and beans – they're nature's fiber patrol, ensuring smooth traffic flow.

- **Sugar Sleuth**: Added sugars lurk in unexpected places – beware the sugary siren song of packaged foods and drinks. Read labels like detective novels, searching for hidden sugars masquerading as "high-fructose corn syrup" or "dextrose."

- **Sweet Alternatives**: Craving a treat? Don't despair! Swap sugary desserts for naturally sweet fruits or low-fat yogurt with a sprinkle of cinnamon. Think gourmet fruit tarts over greasy donuts – your taste buds (and blood sugar) will thank you.

- **Hydration Hero**: Water is the ultimate traffic lubricant. Ditch sugary drinks and sip water regularly. Think of it as keeping your city's water mains flowing, flushing out excess sugar and keeping your energy levels high.

The Balanced Diet Symphony:

A balanced diabetic diet isn't a restrictive prison, it's a vibrant culinary adventure. Explore new, healthy recipes, experiment with spices and herbs, and rediscover the joy of cooking. Think of it as composing your own health symphony, each bite a harmonious note in the overall melody of well-being.

Remember, managing diabetes is a marathon, not a sprint. Don't get discouraged by occasional slip-ups – every healthy choice is a step towards a healthier you. With smart food choices, you can become the architect of your own health, transforming the diabetes-diet dance into a graceful waltz towards a balanced, fulfilling life.

So, ditch the fear of traffic jams and embrace the possibilities. With a little knowledge and a lot of delicious, nutritious choices, you can navigate the complexities of type 2 diabetes and build a thriving city of health within your body.

Chapter 1: 30-Day Meal Plan

Week 1:

Day 1:

- Breakfast: Vegetable Omelette with Spinach and Feta
- Lunch: Grilled Chicken Salad with Lemon Vinaigrette
- Dinner: Baked Cod with Lemon and Herbs
- Snack: Guacamole with Veggie Sticks
- Dessert: Sugar-Free Chocolate Avocado Mousse

Day 2:

- Breakfast: Greek Yogurt Parfait with Berries and Almonds
- Lunch: Quinoa and Black Bean Stuffed Peppers
- Dinner: Roasted Vegetable and Chickpea Bowl
- Snack: Hummus and Whole Grain Crackers
- Dessert: Berry and Almond Crisp

Day 3:

- Breakfast: Avocado and Tomato Breakfast Wrap
- Lunch: Turkey and Vegetable Lettuce Wraps
- Dinner: Beef and Vegetable Stir-Fry
- Snack: Greek Yogurt with Berries and Honey
- Dessert: Greek Yogurt and Berry Popsicles

Day 4:

- Breakfast: Quinoa Breakfast Bowl with Nuts and Seeds
- Lunch: Lentil and Vegetable Soup
- Dinner: Spaghetti Squash with Turkey Bolognese
- Snack: Roasted Chickpeas with Rosemary
- Dessert: Pumpkin Chia Seed Pudding

Day 5:

- Breakfast: Cottage Cheese Pancakes with Sugar-Free Syrup
- Lunch: Grilled Shrimp and Quinoa Salad
- Dinner: Lemon Garlic Herb Grilled Chicken
- Snack: Cheese and Grape Skewers
- Dessert: Baked Apple with Cinnamon and Walnuts

Day 6:

- Breakfast: Chia Seed Pudding with Coconut Milk
- Lunch: Chicken and Vegetable Stir-Fry
- Dinner: Eggplant Parmesan with Whole Grain Pasta
- Snack: Almond and Cranberry Energy Bites
- Dessert: Dark Chocolate-Dipped Strawberries

Day 7:

- Breakfast: Egg Muffins with Turkey and Vegetables
- Lunch: Caprese Salad with Balsamic Glaze
- Dinner: Teriyaki Salmon with Brown Rice
- Snack: Cucumber and Tomato Salsa
- Dessert: Coconut Flour Lemon Bars

Week 2:

Day 8:

- Breakfast: Almond Flour Banana Muffins
- Lunch: Mediterranean Chickpea Salad
- Dinner: Stuffed Bell Peppers with Quinoa and Turkey
- Snack: Hard-Boiled Eggs with Paprika
- Dessert: Almond Flour Banana Bread

Day 9:

- Breakfast: Smoked Salmon and Cream Cheese Bagel Thin
- Lunch: Zucchini Noodles with Pesto and Cherry Tomatoes
- Dinner: Shrimp and Vegetable Skewers
- Snack: Avocado and Black Bean Salsa
- Dessert: Avocado Chocolate Truffles

Day 10:

- Breakfast: Blueberry and Walnut Overnight Oats
- Lunch: Salmon and Asparagus Foil Pack
- Dinner: Sweet Potato and Black Bean Enchiladas
- Snack: Trail Mix with Nuts and Seeds
- Dessert: Blueberry Coconut Ice Cream

Day 11:

- Breakfast: Sweet Potato Hash with Poached Eggs
- Lunch: Turkey and Avocado Wrap
- Dinner: Pesto Zoodles with Grilled Chicken
- Snack: Caprese Bruschetta
- Dessert: Raspberry Cheesecake Bites

Day 12:

- Breakfast: Spinach and Mushroom Frittata
- Lunch: Cauliflower Fried Rice with Tofu
- Dinner: Turkey and Broccoli Casserole
- Snack: Apple Slices with Peanut Butter
- Dessert: Pistachio and Cranberry Bark

Day 13:

- Breakfast: Cinnamon Apple Quinoa Porridge
- Lunch: Tomato Basil Mozzarella Skewers
- Dinner: Mediterranean Baked Chicken
- Snack: Kale Chips with Parmesan
- Dessert: Peach and Berry Sorbet

Day 14:

- Breakfast: Berry Protein Smoothie Bowl
- Lunch: Broccoli and Cheddar Stuffed Chicken Breast
- Dinner: Quinoa and Spinach Stuffed Mushrooms
- Snack: Cottage Cheese with Pineapple
- Dessert: Zucchini Brownies

Week 3:

Day 15:

- Breakfast: Whole Grain Toast with Avocado and Poached Egg
- Lunch: Spinach and Feta Turkey Burger
- Dinner: Sesame Ginger Tofu Stir-Fry
- Snack: Smoked Salmon Cucumber Bites
- Dessert: Vanilla Chia Seed Pudding with Fresh Mango

Day 16:

- Breakfast: Vegetable Omelette with Spinach and Feta
- Lunch: Grilled Chicken Salad with Lemon Vinaigrette
- Dinner: Baked Cod with Lemon and Herbs
- Snack: Guacamole with Veggie Sticks
- Dessert: Sugar-Free Chocolate Avocado Mousse

Day 17:

- Breakfast: Greek Yogurt Parfait with Berries and Almonds

- Lunch: Quinoa and Black Bean Stuffed Peppers

- Dinner: Roasted Vegetable and Chickpea Bowl

- Snack: Hummus and Whole Grain Crackers

- Dessert: Berry and Almond Crisp

Day 18:

- Breakfast: Avocado and Tomato Breakfast Wrap

- Lunch: Turkey and Vegetable Lettuce Wraps

- Dinner: Beef and Vegetable Stir-Fry

- Snack: Greek Yogurt with Berries and Honey

- Dessert: Greek Yogurt and Berry Popsicles

Day 19:

- Breakfast: Quinoa Breakfast Bowl with Nuts and Seeds

- Lunch: Lentil and Vegetable Soup

- Dinner: Spaghetti Squash with Turkey Bolognese

- Snack: Roasted Chickpeas with Rosemary

- Dessert: Pumpkin Chia Seed Pudding

Day 20:

- Breakfast: Cottage Cheese Pancakes with Sugar-Free Syrup
- Lunch: Grilled Shrimp and Quinoa Salad
- Dinner: Lemon Garlic Herb Grilled Chicken
- Snack: Cheese and Grape Skewers
- Dessert: Baked Apple with Cinnamon and Walnuts

Day 21:

- Breakfast: Chia Seed Pudding with Coconut Milk
- Lunch: Chicken and Vegetable Stir-Fry
- Dinner: Eggplant Parmesan with Whole Grain Pasta
- Snack: Almond and Cranberry Energy Bites
- Dessert: Dark Chocolate-Dipped Strawberries

Week 4:

Day 22:

- Breakfast: Almond Flour Banana Muffins
- Lunch: Mediterranean Chickpea Salad
- Dinner: Stuffed Bell Peppers with Quinoa and Turkey
- Snack: Hard-Boiled Eggs with Paprika

- Dessert: Almond Flour Banana Bread

Day 23:

- Breakfast: Smoked Salmon and Cream Cheese Bagel Thin
- Lunch: Zucchini Noodles with Pesto and Cherry Tomatoes
- Dinner: Shrimp and Vegetable Skewers
- Snack: Avocado and Black Bean Salsa
- Dessert: Avocado Chocolate Truffles

Day 24:

- Breakfast: Blueberry and Walnut Overnight Oats
- Lunch: Salmon and Asparagus Foil Pack
- Dinner: Sweet Potato and Black Bean Enchiladas
- Snack: Trail Mix with Nuts and Seeds
- Dessert: Blueberry Coconut Ice Cream

Day 25:

- Breakfast: Sweet Potato Hash with Poached Eggs
- Lunch: Turkey and Avocado Wrap
- Dinner: Pesto Zoodles with Grilled Chicken

- Snack: Caprese Bruschetta
- Dessert: Raspberry Cheesecake Bites

Day 26:

- Breakfast: Spinach and Mushroom Frittata
- Lunch: Cauliflower Fried Rice with Tofu
- Dinner: Turkey and Broccoli Casserole
- Snack: Apple Slices with Peanut Butter
- Dessert: Pistachio and Cranberry Bark

Day 27:

- Breakfast: Cinnamon Apple Quinoa Porridge
- Lunch: Tomato Basil Mozzarella Skewers
- Dinner: Mediterranean Baked Chicken
- Snack: Kale Chips with Parmesan
- Dessert: Peach and Berry Sorbet

Day 28:

- Breakfast: Berry Protein Smoothie Bowl
- Lunch: Broccoli and Cheddar Stuffed Chicken Breast
- Dinner: Quinoa and Spinach Stuffed Mushrooms

- Snack: Cottage Cheese with Pineapple
- Dessert: Zucchini Brownies

Day 29:

- Breakfast: Whole Grain Toast with Avocado and Poached Egg
- Lunch: Spinach and Feta Turkey Burger
- Dinner: Sesame Ginger Tofu Stir-Fry
- Snack: Smoked Salmon Cucumber Bites
- Dessert: Vanilla Chia Seed Pudding with Fresh Mango

Day 30:

- Breakfast: Vegetable Omelette with Spinach and Feta
- Lunch: Grilled Chicken Salad with Lemon Vinaigrette
- Dinner: Baked Cod with Lemon and Herbs
- Snack: Guacamole with Veggie Sticks
- Dessert: Sugar-Free Chocolate Avocado Mousse

Chapter 2: Breakfast Recipes

These recipes are not just nourishing but also bursting with flavor, proving that a diabetic-friendly breakfast can be both delicious and satisfying. Each recipe is crafted with wholesome ingredients, and we've included essential nutrition information to help you make informed choices.

Vegetable Omelette with Spinach and Feta

Ingredients:

- 2 eggs
- 1/4 cup diced bell peppers
- 1/4 cup chopped spinach
- 2 tablespoons crumbled feta cheese
- Salt and pepper to taste

Instructions:

1. In a bowl, whisk the eggs and season with salt and pepper.

2. Heat a non-stick pan over medium heat and add the bell peppers and spinach.

3. Pour the whisked eggs over the vegetables and sprinkle feta cheese on top.

4. Cook until the edges set, then fold the omelette in half.

5. Continue cooking until the omelette is cooked through.

6. Serve hot.

Nutrition Information (per serving):

- Calories: 250
- Protein: 15g
- Carbohydrates: 8g
- Fat: 18g
- Fiber: 2g
- Sugar: 3g
- Portion size: 1 omelette

Greek Yogurt Parfait with Berries and Almonds

Ingredients:

- 1/2 cup Greek yogurt
- 1/4 cup mixed berries (strawberries, blueberries, raspberries)
- 2 tablespoons sliced almonds
- 1 teaspoon honey (optional)

Instructions:

1. In a glass or bowl, layer Greek yogurt, mixed berries, and sliced almonds.
2. Repeat the layers until the container is filled.
3. Drizzle honey on top if desired.
4. Serve chilled.

Nutrition Information (per serving):

- Calories: 180
- Protein: 12g
- Carbohydrates: 15g
- Fat: 8g
- Fiber: 4g

- Sugar: 8g
- Portion size: 1 parfait

Avocado and Tomato Breakfast Wrap

Ingredients:

- 1 whole-grain wrap
- 1/2 avocado, sliced
- 1/2 cup cherry tomatoes, halved
- 1 tablespoon fresh cilantro, chopped
- Salt and pepper to taste

Instructions:

1. Place the sliced avocado in the center of the wrap.
2. Add halved cherry tomatoes on top.
3. Sprinkle with chopped cilantro, salt, and pepper.
4. Fold the sides of the wrap and roll tightly.
5. Slice in half and serve.

Nutrition Information (per serving):

- Calories: 320

- Protein: 8g

- Carbohydrates: 30g

- Fat: 20g

- Fiber: 8g

- Sugar: 3g

- Portion size: 1 wrap

Quinoa Breakfast Bowl with Nuts and Seeds

Ingredients:

- 1/2 cup cooked quinoa

- 2 tablespoons mixed nuts (almonds, walnuts, pistachios)

- 1 tablespoon chia seeds

- 1/2 cup unsweetened almond milk

- 1/2 teaspoon cinnamon

- 1 teaspoon maple syrup (optional)

Instructions:

1. In a bowl, combine cooked quinoa, mixed nuts, and chia seeds.

2. Pour almond milk over the mixture.

3. Sprinkle with cinnamon and drizzle with maple syrup if desired.

4. Stir well and enjoy.

Nutrition Information (per serving):

- Calories: 280
- Protein: 9g
- Carbohydrates: 30g
- Fat: 15g
- Fiber: 6g
- Sugar: 2g
- Portion size: 1 bowl

Cottage Cheese Pancakes with Sugar-Free Syrup

Ingredients:

- 1/2 cup low-fat cottage cheese
- 2 eggs
- 1/4 cup almond flour
- 1/2 teaspoon baking powder

- 1/2 teaspoon vanilla extract
- Sugar-free syrup for topping

Instructions:

1. In a blender, combine cottage cheese, eggs, almond flour, baking powder, and vanilla extract.
2. Blend until smooth.
3. Heat a griddle or non-stick pan over medium heat.
4. Pour small portions of batter onto the griddle and cook until bubbles form.
5. Flip the pancakes and cook until golden brown.
6. Serve with sugar-free syrup.

Nutrition Information (per serving):

- Calories: 220
- Protein: 20g
- Carbohydrates: 8g
- Fat: 12g
- Fiber: 2g
- Sugar: 1g
- Portion size: 3 pancakes

Chia Seed Pudding with Coconut Milk

Ingredients:

- 3 tablespoons chia seeds
- 1 cup unsweetened coconut milk
- 1/2 teaspoon vanilla extract
- 1 tablespoon shredded coconut
- Fresh berries for topping

Instructions:

1. In a bowl, mix chia seeds, coconut milk, and vanilla extract.
2. Refrigerate for at least 4 hours or overnight, allowing the chia seeds to absorb the liquid.
3. Stir the mixture well before serving.
4. Top with shredded coconut and fresh berries.

Nutrition Information (per serving):

- Calories: 180
- Protein: 4g
- Carbohydrates: 15g
- Fat: 12g

- Fiber: 8g
- Sugar: 1g
- Portion size: 1 pudding

Egg Muffins with Turkey and Vegetables

Ingredients:

- 4 large eggs
- 1/2 cup cooked turkey, diced
- 1/2 cup bell peppers, diced
- 1/4 cup spinach, chopped
- Salt and pepper to taste

Instructions:

1. Preheat the oven to 350°F (175°C) and grease a muffin tin.
2. In a bowl, beat the eggs and season with salt and pepper.
3. Stir in diced turkey, bell peppers, and chopped spinach.

4. Pour the mixture into muffin cups, filling each about halfway.

5. Bake for 15-20 minutes or until the eggs are set.

6. Allow to cool slightly before serving.

Nutrition Information (per serving):

- Calories: 150
- Protein: 15g
- Carbohydrates: 2g
- Fat: 9g
- Fiber: 1g
- Sugar: 1g
- Portion size: 2 muffins

Almond Flour Banana Muffins

Ingredients:

- 2 ripe bananas, mashed
- 3 eggs
- 1 cup almond flour
- 1/4 cup coconut oil, melted
- 1 teaspoon baking powder
- 1/2 teaspoon cinnamon

- 1/4 teaspoon salt

Instructions:

1. Preheat the oven to 350°F (175°C) and line a muffin tin with paper liners.
2. In a bowl, combine mashed bananas, eggs, almond flour, melted coconut oil, baking powder, cinnamon, and salt.
3. Mix until well combined.
4. Divide the batter among the muffin cups.
5. Bake for 20-25 minutes or until a toothpick comes out clean.
6. Cool before serving.

Nutrition Information (per serving):

- Calories: 180
- Protein: 6g
- Carbohydrates: 12g
- Fat: 14g
- Fiber: 3g
- Sugar: 6g
- Portion size: 2 muffins

Smoked Salmon and Cream Cheese Bagel Thin

Ingredients:

- 1 whole-grain bagel thin
- 2 tablespoons light cream cheese
- 2 ounces smoked salmon
- Fresh dill for garnish

Instructions:

1. Toast the bagel thin to your liking.
2. Spread light cream cheese on the toasted bagel.
3. Arrange smoked salmon on top.
4. Garnish with fresh dill.

Nutrition Information (per serving):

- Calories: 250
- Protein: 20g
- Carbohydrates: 25g
- Fat: 10g
- Fiber: 4g
- Sugar: 2g
- Portion size: 1 bagel thin

Blueberry and Walnut Overnight Oats

Ingredients:

- 1/2 cup rolled oats
- 1/2 cup unsweetened almond milk
- 1/4 cup blueberries
- 1 tablespoon chopped walnuts
- 1/2 teaspoon vanilla extract
- 1 teaspoon maple syrup (optional)

Instructions:

1. In a jar, combine rolled oats, almond milk, blueberries, chopped walnuts, vanilla extract, and maple syrup if desired.
2. Stir well, cover, and refrigerate overnight.
3. In the morning, give it a good stir and enjoy.

Nutrition Information (per serving):

- Calories: 220
- Protein: 6g
- Carbohydrates: 30g
- Fat: 8g

- Fiber: 6g

- Sugar: 4g

- Portion size: 1 serving

Sweet Potato Hash with Poached Eggs

Ingredients:

- 1 large sweet potato, peeled and grated

- 2 tablespoons olive oil

- 1/2 onion, diced

- 1 bell pepper, diced

- 2 poached eggs

- Salt and pepper to taste

- Fresh parsley for garnish

Instructions:

1. In a skillet, heat olive oil over medium heat.

2. Add grated sweet potato, diced onion, and bell pepper.

3. Sauté until sweet potato is golden and vegetables are tender.

4. Season with salt and pepper.

5. Poach eggs separately and place them on top of the
    sweet potato hash.

6. Garnish with fresh parsley.

Nutrition Information (per serving):

- Calories: 280
- Protein: 10g
- Carbohydrates: 28g
- Fat: 16g
- Fiber: 5g
- Sugar: 8g
- Portion size: 1 serving

Spinach and Mushroom Frittata

Ingredients:

- 4 eggs
- 1/2 cup spinach, chopped
- 1/2 cup mushrooms, sliced
- 1/4 cup feta cheese, crumbled
- Salt and pepper to taste
- 1 tablespoon olive oil

Instructions:

1. Preheat the oven to 350°F (175°C).
2. In a bowl, beat eggs and season with salt and pepper.
3. Heat olive oil in an oven-safe skillet over medium heat.
4. Sauté spinach and mushrooms until wilted.
5. Pour beaten eggs over the vegetables and sprinkle with feta cheese.
6. Transfer the skillet to the oven and bake for 15-20 minutes or until set.
7. Slice and serve.

Nutrition Information (per serving):

- Calories: 220
- Protein: 14g
- Carbohydrates: 6g
- Fat: 16g
- Fiber: 2g
- Sugar: 2g
- Portion size: 1 slice

Cinnamon Apple Quinoa Porridge

Ingredients:

- 1/2 cup cooked quinoa
- 1/2 apple, diced
- 1/4 teaspoon cinnamon
- 1 tablespoon almond butter
- 1 teaspoon honey (optional)

Instructions:

1. In a bowl, combine cooked quinoa, diced apple, cinnamon, almond butter, and honey if desired.
2. Stir until well mixed.
3. Microwave for 1-2 minutes until warm.
4. Serve and enjoy.

Nutrition Information (per serving):

- Calories: 240
- Protein: 7g
- Carbohydrates: 32g
- Fat: 10g
- Fiber: 5g
- Sugar: 8g

- Portion size: 1 serving

Berry Protein Smoothie Bowl

Ingredients:

- 1 cup mixed berries (strawberries, blueberries, raspberries)
- 1/2 banana, frozen
- 1/2 cup Greek yogurt
- 1 scoop protein powder (unflavored or vanilla)
- 1/4 cup almond milk
- Toppings: granola, chia seeds, sliced almonds

Instructions:

1. Blend mixed berries, frozen banana, Greek yogurt, protein powder, and almond milk until smooth.
2. Pour the smoothie into a bowl.
3. Top with granola, chia seeds, and sliced almonds.
4. Serve immediately.

Nutrition Information (per serving):

- Calories: 300
- Protein: 25g

- Carbohydrates: 35g

- Fat: 8g

- Fiber: 8g

- Sugar: 18g

- Portion size: 1 bowl

Whole Grain Toast with Avocado and Poached Egg

Ingredients:

- 1 slice whole-grain bread, toasted

- 1/2 avocado, mashed

- 1 poached egg

- Salt and pepper to taste

- Red pepper flakes for garnish

Instructions:

1. Toast the whole-grain bread to your liking.

2. Spread mashed avocado on the toast.

3. Place a poached egg on top.

4. Season with salt, pepper, and garnish with red pepper flakes.

Nutrition Information (per serving):

- Calories: 220
- Protein: 10g
- Carbohydrates: 20g
- Fat: 12g
- Fiber: 6g
- Sugar: 1g
- Portion size: 1 serving

Chapter 3: Lunch Recipes

These carefully curated recipes emphasize fresh, wholesome ingredients and vibrant flavors, ensuring your midday meal is not only delicious but also supports your overall health. Let's embark on a culinary journey filled with a variety of textures and tastes, from hearty salads to satisfying wraps and savory stir-fries.

Grilled Chicken Salad with Lemon Vinaigrette

Ingredients:

- 1 lb boneless, skinless chicken breasts
- Mixed salad greens (spinach, arugula, and romaine)
- Cherry tomatoes, halved
- Cucumber, sliced
- Red onion, thinly sliced
- Lemon Vinaigrette Dressing

Instructions:

1. Season chicken breasts with salt and pepper, then grill until cooked.

2. Let the chicken rest before slicing it into strips.

3. In a large bowl, combine salad greens, cherry tomatoes, cucumber, and red onion.

4. Top the salad with grilled chicken strips.

5. Drizzle with lemon vinaigrette dressing.

Nutrition Information:

- Calories: 350

- Protein: 30g

- Carbohydrates: 15g

- Fat: 18g

- Fiber: 4g

- Sugar: 3g

- Portion Size: 1 serving

Quinoa and Black Bean Stuffed Peppers

Ingredients:

- Bell peppers (assorted colors)
- Cooked quinoa
- Black beans, drained and rinsed
- Corn kernels
- Diced tomatoes
- Cumin, chili powder, salt, and pepper

Instructions:

1. Preheat the oven to 375°F (190°C).
2. Cut the tops off bell peppers and remove seeds.
3. In a bowl, mix quinoa, black beans, corn, diced tomatoes, and spices.
4. Stuff each pepper with the quinoa mixture.
5. Place stuffed peppers in a baking dish and bake until peppers are tender.

Nutrition Information:

- Calories: 280
- Protein: 12g

- Carbohydrates: 45g
- Fat: 5g
- Fiber: 10g
- Sugar: 5g
- Portion Size: 2 peppers

Turkey and Vegetable Lettuce Wraps

Ingredients:
- Ground turkey
- Lettuce leaves (iceberg or butterhead)
- Carrots, julienned
- Red bell pepper, thinly sliced
- Hoisin sauce, soy sauce, and sesame oil

Instructions:
1. In a skillet, cook ground turkey until browned.
2. Mix in julienned carrots, sliced red bell pepper, hoisin sauce, soy sauce, and sesame oil.
3. Spoon the turkey mixture into lettuce leaves.

4. Roll the leaves into wraps and secure with toothpicks.

Nutrition Information:

- Calories: 220
- Protein: 18g
- Carbohydrates: 10g
- Fat: 12g
- Fiber: 3g
- Sugar: 5g
- Portion Size: 3 wraps

Lentil and Vegetable Soup

Ingredients:

- Green lentils, rinsed
- Carrots, diced
- Celery, chopped
- Onion, finely chopped
- Garlic, minced
- Vegetable broth
- Bay leaves, thyme, salt, and pepper

Instructions:

1. In a large pot, sauté onions, garlic, carrots, and celery until softened.
2. Add green lentils, vegetable broth, bay leaves, thyme, salt, and pepper.
3. Simmer until lentils are tender.
4. Remove bay leaves before serving.

Nutrition Information:

- Calories: 180
- Protein: 12g
- Carbohydrates: 30g
- Fat: 1g
- Fiber: 12g
- Sugar: 5g
- Portion Size: 2 cups

Grilled Shrimp and Quinoa Salad

Ingredients:

- Shrimp, peeled and deveined
- Quinoa, cooked
- Cherry tomatoes, halved

- Cucumber, diced

- Red bell pepper, chopped

- Fresh parsley, chopped

- Olive oil, lemon juice, salt, and pepper

Instructions:

1. Grill shrimp until cooked.

2. In a bowl, combine cooked quinoa, grilled shrimp, tomatoes, cucumber, bell pepper, and parsley.

3. Drizzle with olive oil and lemon juice.

4. Season with salt and pepper.

Nutrition Information:

- Calories: 250

- Protein: 20g

- Carbohydrates: 25g

- Fat: 8g

- Fiber: 4g

- Sugar: 3g

- Portion Size: 1.5 cups

Chicken and Vegetable Stir-Fry

Ingredients:

- Chicken breast, thinly sliced
- Broccoli florets
- Bell peppers (assorted colors), sliced
- Snap peas
- Soy sauce, ginger, garlic, and sesame oil

Instructions:

1. Stir-fry sliced chicken until browned.
2. Add broccoli, bell peppers, and snap peas.
3. Mix in soy sauce, ginger, garlic, and sesame oil.
4. Cook until vegetables are tender.

Nutrition Information:

- Calories: 280
- Protein: 25g
- Carbohydrates: 18g
- Fat: 12g
- Fiber: 6g
- Sugar: 5g
- Portion Size: 1.5 cups

Caprese Salad with Balsamic Glaze

Ingredients:

- Fresh mozzarella cheese, sliced
- Tomatoes, sliced
- Fresh basil leaves
- Balsamic glaze
- Olive oil, salt, and pepper

Instructions:

1. Arrange mozzarella slices, tomato slices, and basil leaves on a serving plate.
2. Drizzle with balsamic glaze and olive oil.
3. Sprinkle with salt and pepper to taste.

Nutrition Information:

- Calories: 220
- Protein: 12g
- Carbohydrates: 6g
- Fat: 18g
- Fiber: 2g
- Sugar: 4g
- Portion Size: 1 cup

Mediterranean Chickpea Salad

Ingredients:

- Chickpeas, drained and rinsed
- Cherry tomatoes, halved
- Cucumber, diced
- Kalamata olives, sliced
- Red onion, finely chopped
- Feta cheese, crumbled
- Olive oil, lemon juice, oregano, salt, and pepper

Instructions:

1. In a bowl, combine chickpeas, tomatoes, cucumber, olives, red onion, and feta cheese.
2. Drizzle with olive oil and lemon juice.
3. Sprinkle with oregano, salt, and pepper.

Nutrition Information:

- Calories: 280
- Protein: 10g
- Carbohydrates: 30g
- Fat: 14g
- Fiber: 8g

- Sugar: 5g
- Portion Size: 1.5 cups

Zucchini Noodles with Pesto and Cherry Tomatoes

Ingredients:

- Zucchini, spiralized
- Cherry tomatoes, halved
- Pesto sauce (homemade or store-bought)
- Pine nuts, toasted

Instructions:

1. Spiralize zucchini into noodles.
2. Toss zucchini noodles with pesto sauce.
3. Add cherry tomatoes and toss until combined.
4. Garnish with toasted pine nuts.

Nutrition Information:

- Calories: 180
- Protein: 5g
- Carbohydrates: 10g

- Fat: 14g

- Fiber: 3g

- Sugar: 5g

- Portion Size: 1.5 cups

Salmon and Asparagus Foil Pack

Ingredients:

- Salmon fillets

- Asparagus spears

- Lemon slices

- Garlic, minced

- Dill, chopped

- Olive oil, salt, and pepper

Instructions:

1. Preheat the oven to 375°F (190°C).

2. Place salmon fillets on foil, surround with asparagus.

3. Drizzle with olive oil, sprinkle minced garlic, dill, salt, and pepper.

4. Seal the foil pack and bake until salmon is cooked through.

Nutrition Information:

- Calories: 320
- Protein: 30g
- Carbohydrates: 8g
- Fat: 20g
- Fiber: 4g
- Sugar: 2g
- Portion Size: 1 fillet with asparagus

Turkey and Avocado Wrap

Ingredients:

- Whole-grain tortilla
- Sliced turkey breast
- Avocado, sliced
- Lettuce leaves
- Tomato, sliced
- Greek yogurt dressing

Instructions:

1. Lay out the tortilla and layer with turkey, avocado, lettuce, and tomato.
2. Drizzle with Greek yogurt dressing.

3. Roll up the wrap and slice before serving.

Nutrition Information:

- Calories: 280
- Protein: 18g
- Carbohydrates: 30g
- Fat: 12g
- Fiber: 8g
- Sugar: 5g
- Portion Size: 1 wrap

Cauliflower Fried Rice with Tofu

Ingredients:

- Cauliflower rice
- Extra-firm tofu, cubed
- Mixed vegetables (peas, carrots, corn)
- Soy sauce, sesame oil, garlic powder
- Green onions, chopped

Instructions:

1. Sauté tofu until golden in sesame oil.
2. Add mixed vegetables and cauliflower rice.

3. Season with soy sauce and garlic powder.

4. Cook until vegetables are tender, garnish with green onions.

Nutrition Information:

- Calories: 250
- Protein: 15g
- Carbohydrates: 20g
- Fat: 14g
- Fiber: 8g
- Sugar: 5g
- Portion Size: 1.5 cups

Tomato Basil Mozzarella Skewers

Ingredients:

- Cherry tomatoes
- Fresh mozzarella balls
- Fresh basil leaves
- Balsamic glaze
- Olive oil, salt, and pepper

Instructions:

1. Thread tomatoes, mozzarella, and basil onto skewers.

2. Drizzle with balsamic glaze and olive oil.

3. Sprinkle with salt and pepper.

Nutrition Information:

- Calories: 180
- Protein: 10g
- Carbohydrates: 6g
- Fat: 14g
- Fiber: 2g
- Sugar: 3g
- Portion Size: 4 skewers

Broccoli and Cheddar Stuffed Chicken Breast

Ingredients:

- Chicken breast
- Broccoli florets, steamed
- Cheddar cheese, shredded

- Garlic powder, paprika, salt, and pepper

Instructions:

1. Butterfly chicken breast and season with garlic powder, paprika, salt, and pepper.
2. Stuff with steamed broccoli and cheddar cheese.
3. Bake until chicken is cooked and cheese is melted.

Nutrition Information:

- Calories: 280
- Protein: 30g
- Carbohydrates: 8g
- Fat: 14g
- Fiber: 4g
- Sugar: 2g
- Portion Size: 1 stuffed breast

Spinach and Feta Turkey Burger

Ingredients:

- Ground turkey
- Fresh spinach, chopped
- Feta cheese, crumbled

- Whole-grain burger buns
- Tzatziki sauce

Instructions:

1. Mix ground turkey, chopped spinach, and crumbled feta.
2. Form into burger patties and grill until cooked.
3. Serve on whole-grain buns with tzatziki sauce.

Nutrition Information:

- Calories: 320
- Protein: 25g
- Carbohydrates: 25g
- Fat: 15g
- Fiber: 4g
- Sugar: 3g
- Portion Size: 1 burger

Chapter 4: Dinner Recipes

These recipes are crafted to meet the dietary needs of individuals with type 2 diabetes while offering a delightful dining experience. Each dish is thoughtfully prepared, combining wholesome ingredients and flavors that make managing your blood sugar levels a delicious journey.

Baked Cod with Lemon and Herbs

Ingredients:

- 4 cod fillets
- 2 tablespoons olive oil
- 1 lemon (juiced and zested)
- 2 cloves garlic (minced)
- 1 tablespoon fresh parsley (chopped)
- Salt and pepper to taste

Instructions:

1. Preheat the oven to 375°F (190°C).
2. Place cod fillets on a baking sheet.

3. In a bowl, mix olive oil, lemon juice, lemon zest, minced garlic, chopped parsley, salt, and pepper.

4. Pour the mixture over cod fillets, ensuring they are evenly coated.

5. Bake for 15-20 minutes or until the fish flakes easily with a fork.

6. Serve with a side of steamed vegetables.

Nutrition Information:

- Calories: 250
- Protein: 30g
- Carbohydrates: 3g
- Fat: 12g
- Fiber: 1g
- Sugar: 1g
- Portion Size: 1 fillet

Roasted Vegetable and Chickpea Bowl

Ingredients:

- 1 cup chickpeas (cooked)

- 2 cups mixed vegetables (bell peppers, zucchini, cherry tomatoes)
- 2 tablespoons olive oil
- 1 teaspoon cumin
- 1 teaspoon paprika
- Salt and pepper to taste

Instructions:

1. Preheat the oven to 400°F (200°C).
2. Toss chickpeas and vegetables with olive oil, cumin, paprika, salt, and pepper.
3. Spread the mixture on a baking sheet.
4. Roast for 25-30 minutes or until vegetables are tender.
5. Serve over a bed of quinoa or brown rice.

Nutrition Information:

- Calories: 300
- Protein: 10g
- Carbohydrates: 45g
- Fat: 12g
- Fiber: 12g

- Sugar: 8g
- Portion Size: 1 bowl

Beef and Vegetable Stir-Fry

Ingredients:

- 1 pound lean beef strips
- 2 cups mixed stir-fry vegetables (broccoli, bell peppers, snap peas)
- 2 tablespoons soy sauce (low-sodium)
- 1 tablespoon sesame oil
- 1 teaspoon ginger (minced)
- 2 cloves garlic (minced)
- Brown rice for serving

Instructions:

1. In a wok or skillet, heat sesame oil over medium-high heat.
2. Add beef strips and stir-fry until browned.
3. Add minced ginger and garlic, stir-frying for another minute.
4. Toss in the mixed vegetables and soy sauce, cooking until vegetables are crisp-tender.

5. Serve over a bed of brown rice.

Nutrition Information:

- Calories: 350
- Protein: 25g
- Carbohydrates: 30g
- Fat: 15g
- Fiber: 5g
- Sugar: 3g
- Portion Size: 1 cup

Spaghetti Squash with Turkey Bolognese

Ingredients:

- 1 medium spaghetti squash
- 1 pound ground turkey
- 1 onion (diced)
- 2 cloves garlic (minced)
- 1 can crushed tomatoes (low-sugar)
- 1 teaspoon Italian seasoning
- Salt and pepper to taste

Instructions:

1. Preheat the oven to 375°F (190°C).

2. Cut the spaghetti squash in half and remove seeds.

3. Place the halves face down on a baking sheet and bake for 40-45 minutes.

4. In a skillet, brown ground turkey with diced onion and minced garlic.

5. Add crushed tomatoes, Italian seasoning, salt, and pepper, simmering for 15 minutes.

6. Scrape the spaghetti squash strands with a fork and top with turkey bolognese.

Nutrition Information:

- Calories: 320
- Protein: 22g
- Carbohydrates: 30g
- Fat: 14g
- Fiber: 8g
- Sugar: 10g
- Portion Size: 1 bowl

Lemon Garlic Herb Grilled Chicken

Ingredients:

- 4 boneless, skinless chicken breasts
- 2 tablespoons olive oil
- 1 lemon (juiced)
- 3 cloves garlic (minced)
- 1 teaspoon dried herbs (rosemary, thyme, oregano)
- Salt and pepper to taste

Instructions:

1. Preheat the grill to medium-high heat.
2. In a bowl, mix olive oil, lemon juice, minced garlic, dried herbs, salt, and pepper.
3. Marinate chicken breasts in the mixture for at least 30 minutes.
4. Grill chicken for 6-8 minutes per side or until fully cooked.
5. Let it rest before slicing and serve with steamed vegetables.

Nutrition Information:

- Calories: 280

- Protein: 30g

- Carbohydrates: 2g

- Fat: 16g

- Fiber: 0g

- Sugar: 0g

- Portion Size: 1 chicken breast

Eggplant Parmesan with Whole Grain Pasta

Ingredients:

- 1 large eggplant (sliced)

- 1 cup whole grain pasta

- 1 cup tomato sauce (low-sugar)

- 1 cup mozzarella cheese (shredded)

- 1/4 cup Parmesan cheese (grated)

- 1 teaspoon dried basil

- 1 teaspoon dried oregano

Instructions:

1. Preheat the oven to 375°F (190°C).

2. Arrange eggplant slices on a baking sheet and bake for 15-20 minutes.

3. Cook whole grain pasta according to package instructions.

4. In a baking dish, layer eggplant slices, tomato sauce, mozzarella, and Parmesan.

5. Repeat the layers and sprinkle dried basil and oregano on top.

6. Bake for 25-30 minutes or until cheese is bubbly and golden.

Nutrition Information:

- Calories: 340
- Protein: 18g
- Carbohydrates: 40g
- Fat: 14g
- Fiber: 10g
- Sugar: 5g
- Portion Size: 1 serving

Teriyaki Salmon with Brown Rice

Ingredients:

- 4 salmon fillets
- 1/4 cup low-sodium teriyaki sauce
- 2 tablespoons honey
- 1 tablespoon sesame seeds
- 2 cups cooked brown rice
- Green onions (sliced, for garnish)

Instructions:

1. In a bowl, mix teriyaki sauce, honey, and sesame seeds.
2. Marinate salmon fillets in the mixture for 20 minutes.
3. Grill or bake salmon until cooked through.
4. Serve over a bed of brown rice, garnished with sliced green onions.

Nutrition Information:

- Calories: 380
- Protein: 25g
- Carbohydrates: 40g
- Fat: 15g

- Fiber: 3g

- Sugar: 10g

- Portion Size: 1 fillet with rice

Stuffed Bell Peppers with Quinoa and Turkey

Ingredients:

- 4 bell peppers (halved and seeds removed)

- 1 cup quinoa (cooked)

- 1/2 pound ground turkey

- 1 cup black beans (canned, drained)

- 1 cup diced tomatoes

- 1 teaspoon cumin

- 1 teaspoon chili powder

- Salt and pepper to taste

Instructions:

1. Preheat the oven to 375°F (190°C).

2. In a skillet, brown ground turkey and season with cumin, chili powder, salt, and pepper.

3. In a bowl, mix cooked quinoa, black beans, diced tomatoes, and the cooked turkey.

4. Stuff bell pepper halves with the mixture and bake for 25-30 minutes.

Nutrition Information:

- Calories: 320
- Protein: 22g
- Carbohydrates: 40g
- Fat: 8g
- Fiber: 8g
- Sugar: 5g
- Portion Size: 2 pepper halves

Shrimp and Vegetable Skewers

Ingredients:

- 1 pound shrimp (peeled and deveined)
- 2 bell peppers (cut into chunks)
- 1 zucchini (sliced)
- 1 red onion (cut into wedges)
- 2 tablespoons olive oil
- 1 tablespoon lemon juice

- 1 teaspoon smoked paprika
- Salt and pepper to taste

Instructions:

1. Preheat the grill or grill pan.
2. In a bowl, mix olive oil, lemon juice, smoked paprika, salt, and pepper.
3. Thread shrimp, bell peppers, zucchini, and red onion onto skewers.
4. Brush skewers with the olive oil mixture.
5. Grill for 3-4 minutes per side or until shrimp are opaque.
6. Serve with a side of quinoa or a green salad.

Nutrition Information:

- Calories: 250
- Protein: 20g
- Carbohydrates: 15g
- Fat: 12g
- Fiber: 4g
- Sugar: 6g
- Portion Size: 1 skewer

Sweet Potato and Black Bean Enchiladas

Ingredients:

- 2 medium sweet potatoes (peeled and diced)
- 1 can black beans (low-sodium, drained)
- 1 cup corn kernels (fresh or frozen)
- 1 teaspoon cumin
- 1 teaspoon chili powder
- 8 whole wheat tortillas
- 1 cup enchilada sauce (low-sugar)
- 1 cup shredded cheddar cheese

Instructions:

1. Preheat the oven to 375°F (190°C).
2. Steam or roast sweet potatoes until tender.
3. In a bowl, mix sweet potatoes, black beans, corn, cumin, and chili powder.
4. Spoon the mixture into tortillas and roll them up.
5. Place the enchiladas in a baking dish, top with enchilada sauce and cheese.
6. Bake for 20-25 minutes or until the cheese is melted and bubbly.

Nutrition Information:

- Calories: 380
- Protein: 15g
- Carbohydrates: 60g
- Fat: 10g
- Fiber: 10g
- Sugar: 8g
- Portion Size: 2 enchiladas

Pesto Zoodles with Grilled Chicken

Ingredients:

- 2 zucchinis (spiralized into noodles)
- 1 pound chicken breasts (grilled and sliced)
- 1/2 cup cherry tomatoes (halved)
- 1/4 cup pesto sauce
- 2 tablespoons pine nuts (toasted)
- Fresh basil leaves for garnish

Instructions:

1. In a pan, sauté zucchini noodles until just tender.
2. Toss the zoodles with grilled chicken, cherry tomatoes, and pesto sauce.

3. Sprinkle toasted pine nuts on top.

4. Garnish with fresh basil leaves before serving.

Nutrition Information:

- Calories: 320

- Protein: 30g

- Carbohydrates: 10g

- Fat: 18g

- Fiber: 3g

- Sugar: 4g

- Portion Size: 1 serving

Turkey and Broccoli Casserole

Ingredients:

- 1 pound ground turkey

- 2 cups broccoli florets

- 1 cup quinoa (cooked)

- 1 cup low-fat cheddar cheese (shredded)

- 1/2 cup plain Greek yogurt

- 1 teaspoon garlic powder

- Salt and pepper to taste

Instructions:

1. Preheat the oven to 375°F (190°C).

2. In a skillet, brown ground turkey with garlic powder, salt, and pepper.

3. In a large bowl, combine cooked quinoa, broccoli, turkey, Greek yogurt, and half of the shredded cheese.

4. Transfer the mixture to a baking dish, top with the remaining cheese, and bake for 25-30 minutes.

Nutrition Information:

- Calories: 350
- Protein: 25g
- Carbohydrates: 30g
- Fat: 15g
- Fiber: 5g
- Sugar: 3g
- Portion Size: 1 serving

Mediterranean Baked Chicken

Ingredients:

- 4 boneless, skinless chicken thighs

- 1 cup cherry tomatoes (halved)
- 1/2 cup Kalamata olives (pitted)
- 1/4 cup feta cheese (crumbled)
- 2 tablespoons olive oil
- 1 teaspoon dried oregano
- 1 teaspoon garlic powder
- Salt and pepper to taste

Instructions:

1. Preheat the oven to 400°F (200°C).
2. Season chicken thighs with dried oregano, garlic powder, salt, and pepper.
3. Place chicken in a baking dish and surround with cherry tomatoes and Kalamata olives.
4. Drizzle olive oil over the chicken and vegetables.
5. Bake for 25-30 minutes or until chicken is cooked through.
6. Sprinkle crumbled feta over the top before serving.

Nutrition Information:

- Calories: 380
- Protein: 30g

- Carbohydrates: 8g

- Fat: 25g

- Fiber: 2g

- Sugar: 3g

- Portion Size: 1 chicken thigh

Quinoa and Spinach Stuffed Mushrooms

Ingredients:

- 16 large mushrooms (cleaned and stems removed)

- 1 cup cooked quinoa

- 1 cup fresh spinach (chopped)

- 1/4 cup grated Parmesan cheese

- 2 cloves garlic (minced)

- 2 tablespoons olive oil

- Salt and pepper to taste

Instructions:

1. Preheat the oven to 375°F (190°C).

2. In a skillet, sauté garlic and spinach in olive oil until wilted.

3. In a bowl, mix quinoa, sautéed spinach, and Parmesan cheese.

4. Stuff each mushroom with the quinoa mixture.

5. Bake for 20-25 minutes or until mushrooms are tender.

Nutrition Information:

- Calories: 180
- Protein: 8g
- Carbohydrates: 20g
- Fat: 8g
- Fiber: 4g
- Sugar: 2g
- Portion Size: 4 mushrooms

Sesame Ginger Tofu Stir-Fry

Ingredients:

- 1 block extra-firm tofu (pressed and cubed)
- 2 cups broccoli florets
- 1 red bell pepper (sliced)
- 1 cup snap peas
- 2 tablespoons soy sauce (low-sodium)

- 1 tablespoon sesame oil
- 1 tablespoon rice vinegar
- 1 tablespoon maple syrup
- 1 teaspoon fresh ginger (grated)
- 2 cloves garlic (minced)
- 1 tablespoon sesame seeds (toasted)
- Green onions for garnish

Instructions:

1. In a wok or skillet, heat sesame oil over medium-high heat.
2. Add cubed tofu and stir-fry until golden brown.
3. Add broccoli, bell pepper, and snap peas, continuing to stir-fry until vegetables are crisp-tender.
4. In a small bowl, mix soy sauce, rice vinegar, maple syrup, ginger, and garlic.
5. Pour the sauce over the tofu and vegetables, tossing to coat evenly.
6. Sprinkle toasted sesame seeds and garnish with green onions before serving.

Nutrition Information:

- Calories: 280
- Protein: 18g
- Carbohydrates: 20g
- Fat: 15g
- Fiber: 6g
- Sugar: 8g
- Portion Size: 1 serving

Chapter 5: Snacks and Appetizers

In this chapter, we present an array of delectable and wholesome options that cater to your craving for flavor without compromising your health. Each recipe is crafted to bring joy to your snack time while maintaining a balance of essential nutrients.

Guacamole with Veggie Sticks

Ingredients:

- 2 ripe avocados
- 1 medium tomato, diced
- 1/4 cup red onion, finely chopped
- 1 clove garlic, minced
- 1 lime, juiced
- Salt and pepper to taste
- Carrot and cucumber sticks for dipping

Instructions:

1. Mash avocados in a bowl.

2. Add diced tomato, chopped red onion, minced garlic, lime juice, salt, and pepper. Mix well.

3. Serve with carrot and cucumber sticks.

Nutrition Information:

- Calories: 120
- Protein: 2g
- Carbohydrates: 7g
- Fat: 10g
- Fiber: 5g
- Sugar: 1g
- Portion Size: 1/4 cup guacamole with veggie sticks

Hummus and Whole Grain Crackers

Ingredients:

- 1 can (15 oz) chickpeas, drained
- 1/4 cup tahini
- 1/4 cup olive oil
- 1 clove garlic, minced
- 1 lemon, juiced
- Salt and cumin to taste
- Whole grain crackers for serving

Instructions:

1. Blend chickpeas, tahini, olive oil, minced garlic, lemon juice, salt, and cumin until smooth.
2. Serve with whole grain crackers.

Nutrition Information:

- Calories: 140
- Protein: 4g
- Carbohydrates: 12g
- Fat: 9g
- Fiber: 3g
- Sugar: 1g
- Portion Size: 2 tablespoons hummus with crackers

Greek Yogurt with Berries and Honey

Ingredients:

- 1 cup Greek yogurt
- Mixed berries (strawberries, blueberries, raspberries)
- 1 tablespoon honey

Instructions:

1. Spoon Greek yogurt into a bowl.

2. Top with mixed berries and drizzle honey over the
    top.

Nutrition Information:

- Calories: 180

- Protein: 15g

- Carbohydrates: 20g

- Fat: 5g

- Fiber: 2g

- Sugar: 15g

- Portion Size: 1 cup Greek yogurt with berries and
  honey

Roasted Chickpeas with Rosemary

Ingredients:

- 1 can (15 oz) chickpeas, drained and rinsed

- 1 tablespoon olive oil

- 1 teaspoon dried rosemary

- Salt and cayenne pepper to taste

Instructions:

1. Preheat oven to 400°F (200°C).

2. Toss chickpeas with olive oil, dried rosemary, salt, and cayenne pepper.

3. Roast in the oven for 25-30 minutes until crispy.

Nutrition Information:

- Calories: 120

- Protein: 5g

- Carbohydrates: 15g

- Fat: 4g

- Fiber: 4g

- Sugar: 3g

- Portion Size: 1/2 cup roasted chickpeas

Cheese and Grape Skewers

Ingredients:

- Cubes of your favorite cheese (cheddar, mozzarella, or feta)

- Red and green grapes

Instructions:

1. Thread cheese cubes and grapes onto skewers alternately.

Nutrition Information:

- Calories: 150
- Protein: 7g
- Carbohydrates: 10g
- Fat: 9g
- Fiber: 1g
- Sugar: 7g
- Portion Size: 5 skewers

Almond and Cranberry Energy Bites

Ingredients:

- 1 cup rolled oats
- 1/2 cup almond butter
- 1/4 cup honey
- 1/2 cup dried cranberries
- 1/4 cup chopped almonds
- 1 teaspoon vanilla extract

Instructions:

1. Mix rolled oats, almond butter, honey, dried cranberries, chopped almonds, and vanilla extract in a bowl.

2. Form into small energy bites and refrigerate for at least 30 minutes.

Nutrition Information:

- Calories: 90
- Protein: 3g
- Carbohydrates: 12g
- Fat: 4g
- Fiber: 2g
- Sugar: 6g
- Portion Size: 2 energy bites

Cucumber and Tomato Salsa

Ingredients:

- 1 cucumber, diced
- 1 cup cherry tomatoes, halved
- 1/4 cup red onion, finely chopped
- 1/4 cup fresh cilantro, chopped

- 1 lime, juiced
- Salt and pepper to taste

Instructions:

1. Combine diced cucumber, cherry tomatoes, red onion, cilantro, lime juice, salt, and pepper in a bowl.
2. Mix well and refrigerate before serving.

Nutrition Information:

- Calories: 40
- Protein: 1g
- Carbohydrates: 8g
- Fat: 1g
- Fiber: 2g
- Sugar: 3g
- Portion Size: 1/2 cup salsa

Hard-Boiled Eggs with Paprika

Ingredients:

- Hard-boiled eggs
- Paprika
- Salt and pepper to taste

Instructions:

1. Slice hard-boiled eggs in half.

2. Sprinkle with paprika, salt, and pepper.

Nutrition Information:

- Calories: 70

- Protein: 6g

- Carbohydrates: 1g

- Fat: 5g

- Fiber: 0g

- Sugar: 0g

- Portion Size: 2 halves

Avocado and Black Bean Salsa

Ingredients:

- 1 ripe avocado, diced

- 1 can (15 oz) black beans, drained and rinsed

- 1/4 cup red onion, finely chopped

- 1/4 cup cilantro, chopped

- 1 lime, juiced

- Salt and cumin to taste

Instructions:

1. In a bowl, combine diced avocado, black beans, red onion, cilantro, lime juice, salt, and cumin.

2. Mix well and refrigerate.

Nutrition Information:

- Calories: 150
- Protein: 6g
- Carbohydrates: 20g
- Fat: 7g
- Fiber: 8g
- Sugar: 1g
- Portion Size: 1/2 cup salsa

Trail Mix with Nuts and Seeds

Ingredients:

- Almonds, walnuts, pumpkin seeds, sunflower seeds, and dried cranberries

Instructions:

1. Mix almonds, walnuts, pumpkin seeds, sunflower seeds, and dried cranberries in a bowl.

2. Portion into small snack-sized bags.

Nutrition Information:

- Calories: 180
- Protein: 6g
- Carbohydrates: 12g
- Fat: 13g
- Fiber: 3g
- Sugar: 6g
- Portion Size: 1/4 cup trail mix

Caprese Bruschetta

Ingredients:

- Cherry tomatoes, halved
- Fresh mozzarella, diced
- Fresh basil leaves, chopped
- Balsamic glaze
- Baguette slices

Instructions:

1. Combine cherry tomatoes, fresh mozzarella, and chopped basil in a bowl.

2. Spoon the mixture onto baguette slices and drizzle with balsamic glaze.

Nutrition Information:

- Calories: 120
- Protein: 5g
- Carbohydrates: 15g
- Fat: 5g
- Fiber: 1g
- Sugar: 2g
- Portion Size: 3 bruschetta slices

Apple Slices with Peanut Butter

Ingredients:

- Apple slices
- Natural peanut butter

Instructions:

1. Spread peanut butter on apple slices.

Nutrition Information:

- Calories: 160

- Protein: 4g

- Carbohydrates: 18g

- Fat: 9g

- Fiber: 4g

- Sugar: 12g

- Portion Size: 1 medium apple with 2 tablespoons peanut butter

Kale Chips with Parmesan

Ingredients:

- Fresh kale, stems removed and torn into pieces
- Olive oil
- Grated Parmesan cheese
- Salt and pepper to taste

Instructions:

1. Preheat oven to 350°F (175°C).

2. Toss kale pieces with olive oil, Parmesan cheese, salt, and pepper.

3. Bake for 10-15 minutes until crispy.

Nutrition Information:

- Calories: 90
- Protein: 4g
- Carbohydrates: 7g
- Fat: 6g
- Fiber: 2g
- Sugar: 1g
- Portion Size: 1 cup kale chips

Cottage Cheese with Pineapple

Ingredients:

- Low-fat cottage cheese
- Fresh pineapple chunks

Instructions:

1. Combine cottage cheese and fresh pineapple chunks in a bowl.

Nutrition Information:

- Calories: 120
- Protein: 14g
- Carbohydrates: 15g

- Fat: 2g

- Fiber: 1g

- Sugar: 11g

- Portion Size: 1 cup cottage cheese with pineapple

Smoked Salmon Cucumber Bites

Ingredients:

- Cucumber slices

- Smoked salmon

- Cream cheese

- Fresh dill

Instructions:

1. Spread cream cheese on cucumber slices.

2. Top with smoked salmon and garnish with fresh dill.

Nutrition Information:

- Calories: 90

- Protein: 6g

- Carbohydrates: 2g

- Fat: 6g

- Fiber: 0g

- Sugar: 1g
- Portion Size: 5 bites

Chapter 6: Desserts

These recipes prioritize flavor without compromising on health, offering a sweet treat after meals that aligns with a diabetic-friendly lifestyle. From creamy indulgences to fruity delights, each dessert is designed with your well-being in mind.

Sugar-Free Chocolate Avocado Mousse

Ingredients:

- 2 ripe avocados
- 1/3 cup unsweetened cocoa powder
- 1/4 cup sugar-free sweetener
- 1/4 cup almond milk
- 1 teaspoon vanilla extract
- Pinch of salt

Instructions:

1. Blend avocados, cocoa powder, sweetener, almond milk, vanilla extract, and a pinch of salt until smooth.

2. Refrigerate for at least 2 hours.

3. Serve in small portions.

Nutrition Information (per serving):

- Calories: 120
- Protein: 2g
- Carbohydrates: 8g
- Fat: 10g
- Fiber: 5g
- Sugar: 1g
- Portion size: 1/2 cup

Berry and Almond Crisp

Ingredients:

- 2 cups mixed berries (strawberries, blueberries, raspberries)
- 1/2 cup almond flour
- 1/4 cup chopped almonds
- 2 tablespoons sugar-free sweetener
- 1 teaspoon cinnamon
- 2 tablespoons melted butter (unsalted)

Instructions:

1. Mix berries with sweetener and spread in a baking dish.
2. Combine almond flour, chopped almonds, sweetener, cinnamon, and melted butter. Sprinkle over berries.
3. Bake at 350°F (175°C) for 25-30 minutes until golden.

Nutrition Information (per serving):

- Calories: 150
- Protein: 4g
- Carbohydrates: 12g
- Fat: 10g
- Fiber: 5g
- Sugar: 4g
- Portion size: 1/2 cup

Greek Yogurt and Berry Popsicles

Ingredients:

- 1 cup Greek yogurt (unsweetened)
- 1 cup mixed berries

- 2 tablespoons sugar-free sweetener

- 1 teaspoon vanilla extract

Instructions:

1. Blend yogurt, berries, sweetener, and vanilla extract until smooth.
2. Pour into popsicle molds and freeze for 4-6 hours.
3. Enjoy a refreshing popsicle guilt-free.

Nutrition Information (per serving):

- Calories: 80
- Protein: 5g
- Carbohydrates: 10g
- Fat: 2g
- Fiber: 3g
- Sugar: 5g
- Portion size: 1 popsicle

Pumpkin Chia Seed Pudding

Ingredients:

- 1/2 cup canned pumpkin puree
- 2 tablespoons chia seeds

- 1 cup unsweetened almond milk
- 1/4 cup sugar-free sweetener
- 1/2 teaspoon pumpkin spice

Instructions:

1. Mix pumpkin puree, chia seeds, almond milk, sweetener, and pumpkin spice in a bowl.
2. Refrigerate for at least 4 hours or overnight.
3. Stir well before serving.

Nutrition Information (per serving):

- Calories: 90
- Protein: 3g
- Carbohydrates: 10g
- Fat: 5g
- Fiber: 7g
- Sugar: 1g
- Portion size: 1/2 cup

Baked Apple with Cinnamon and Walnuts

Ingredients:

- 2 apples, cored and sliced
- 1 tablespoon lemon juice
- 1 teaspoon cinnamon
- 2 tablespoons chopped walnuts
- 1 tablespoon sugar-free sweetener

Instructions:

1. Toss apple slices with lemon juice, cinnamon, walnuts, and sweetener.
2. Bake at 375°F (190°C) for 20-25 minutes until apples are tender.

Nutrition Information (per serving):

- Calories: 120
- Protein: 1g
- Carbohydrates: 18g
- Fat: 6g
- Fiber: 5g
- Sugar: 10g

- Portion size: 1/2 apple

Dark Chocolate-Dipped Strawberries

Ingredients:

- 1 cup fresh strawberries
- 1/4 cup dark chocolate (at least 70% cocoa)
- 1 tablespoon chopped nuts (optional)

Instructions:

1. Melt dark chocolate in a microwave-safe bowl.
2. Dip each strawberry into the melted chocolate, coating halfway.
3. Place on parchment paper and sprinkle with chopped nuts if desired.
4. Refrigerate until the chocolate hardens.

Nutrition Information (per serving):

- Calories: 60
- Protein: 1g
- Carbohydrates: 10g
- Fat: 4g
- Fiber: 2g

- Sugar: 6g
- Portion size: 4 strawberries

Coconut Flour Lemon Bars

Ingredients:

- 1/2 cup coconut flour
- 1/4 cup almond flour
- 1/4 cup melted coconut oil
- 2 tablespoons sugar-free sweetener
- Zest and juice of 2 lemons
- 4 eggs

Instructions:

1. Mix coconut flour, almond flour, melted coconut oil, sweetener, lemon zest, lemon juice, and eggs.
2. Bake at 350°F (175°C) for 20-25 minutes until set.
3. Cool and cut into bars.

Nutrition Information (per serving):

- Calories: 90
- Protein: 3g
- Carbohydrates: 6g

- Fat: 6g

- Fiber: 3g

- Sugar: 1g

- Portion size: 1 bar

Almond Flour Banana Bread

Ingredients:

- 2 ripe bananas, mashed

- 1 cup almond flour

- 1/4 cup coconut flour

- 3 eggs

- 1/4 cup melted coconut oil

- 1 teaspoon vanilla extract

- 1/2 teaspoon baking soda

- 1/4 teaspoon salt

Instructions:

1. Mix mashed bananas, almond flour, coconut flour, eggs, melted coconut oil, vanilla extract, baking soda, and salt.

2. Pour into a greased loaf pan.

3. Bake at 350°F (175°C) for 40-45 minutes or until a toothpick comes out clean.

Nutrition Information (per serving):

- Calories: 120
- Protein: 4g
- Carbohydrates: 10g
- Fat: 8g
- Fiber: 3g
- Sugar: 4g
- Portion size: 1 slice

Avocado Chocolate Truffles

Ingredients:

- 1 ripe avocado
- 1/4 cup unsweetened cocoa powder
- 2 tablespoons almond flour
- 2 tablespoons sugar-free sweetener
- 1/2 teaspoon vanilla extract
- Dash of salt
- Shredded coconut or chopped nuts for coating

Instructions:

1. Mash avocado and mix with cocoa powder, almond flour, sweetener, vanilla extract, and salt.
2. Refrigerate for 30 minutes.
3. Form into small truffles and roll in shredded coconut or chopped nuts.

Nutrition Information (per serving):

- Calories: 60
- Protein: 2g
- Carbohydrates: 5g
- Fat: 4g
- Fiber: 3g
- Sugar: 0g
- Portion size: 2 truffles

Blueberry Coconut Ice Cream

Ingredients:

- 2 cups frozen blueberries
- 1 can (14 oz) coconut milk (full-fat)
- 1/4 cup sugar-free sweetener
- 1 teaspoon vanilla extract

Instructions:

1. Blend blueberries, coconut milk, sweetener, and vanilla extract until smooth.

2. Freeze in an airtight container for at least 4 hours.

3. Scoop and serve.

Nutrition Information (per serving):

- Calories: 120
- Protein: 1g
- Carbohydrates: 15g
- Fat: 7g
- Fiber: 3g
- Sugar: 8g
- Portion size: 1/2 cup

Raspberry Cheesecake Bites

Ingredients:

- 1 cup fresh raspberries
- 1/2 cup cream cheese (softened)
- 2 tablespoons sugar-free sweetener
- 1 teaspoon vanilla extract

Instructions:

1. In a bowl, mix cream cheese, sweetener, and vanilla extract until smooth.
2. Gently fold in fresh raspberries.
3. Spoon mixture into mini muffin cups and freeze for 2 hours.

Nutrition Information (per serving):

- Calories: 90
- Protein: 2g
- Carbohydrates: 5g
- Fat: 7g
- Fiber: 2g
- Sugar: 2g
- Portion size: 2 bites

Pistachio and Cranberry Bark

Ingredients:

- 1/2 cup shelled pistachios
- 1/4 cup dried cranberries (unsweetened)
- 1/4 cup dark chocolate (at least 70% cocoa)

Instructions:

1. Melt dark chocolate and spread on a parchment-lined tray.

2. Sprinkle pistachios and cranberries over the chocolate.

3. Refrigerate until set and break into pieces.

Nutrition Information (per serving):

- Calories: 80
- Protein: 2g
- Carbohydrates: 8g
- Fat: 5g
- Fiber: 2g
- Sugar: 4g
- Portion size: 2 squares

Peach and Berry Sorbet

Ingredients:

- 2 cups frozen peaches
- 1 cup mixed berries
- 1/4 cup sugar-free sweetener
- 1 tablespoon lemon juice

Instructions:

1. Blend frozen peaches, mixed berries, sweetener, and lemon juice until smooth.

2. Freeze in a shallow container for at least 3 hours.

3. Scoop and enjoy.

Nutrition Information (per serving):

- Calories: 70

- Protein: 1g

- Carbohydrates: 15g

- Fat: 1g

- Fiber: 3g

- Sugar: 9g

- Portion size: 1/2 cup

Zucchini Brownies

Ingredients:

- 1 cup shredded zucchini

- 1/2 cup almond flour

- 1/4 cup cocoa powder

- 1/4 cup sugar-free sweetener

- 2 eggs

- 1/4 cup melted coconut oil

- 1 teaspoon vanilla extract

- 1/2 teaspoon baking powder

- Pinch of salt

Instructions:

1. Mix shredded zucchini, almond flour, cocoa powder, sweetener, eggs, melted coconut oil, vanilla extract, baking powder, and salt.

2. Spread into a baking pan and bake at 350°F (175°C) for 25-30 minutes.

Nutrition Information (per serving):

- Calories: 100

- Protein: 3g

- Carbohydrates: 8g

- Fat: 7g

- Fiber: 3g

- Sugar: 2g

- Portion size: 1 square

Vanilla Chia Seed Pudding with Fresh Mango

Ingredients:

- 1/4 cup chia seeds
- 1 cup unsweetened almond milk
- 1 tablespoon sugar-free sweetener
- 1 teaspoon vanilla extract
- 1/2 cup fresh mango, diced

Instructions:

1. Mix chia seeds, almond milk, sweetener, and vanilla extract in a jar.
2. Refrigerate for at least 4 hours or overnight.
3. Top with fresh mango before serving.

Nutrition Information (per serving):

- Calories: 80
- Protein: 2g
- Carbohydrates: 10g
- Fat: 4g
- Fiber: 6g
- Sugar: 3g
- Portion size: 1/2 cup

Chapter 7: Smoothies

These smoothies are not only delicious but also packed with wholesome ingredients to support your overall well-being. From the Green Power Smoothie with Spinach and Kale to the Raspberry Coconut Water Electrolyte Smoothie, each recipe brings a unique combination of flavors and nutrients.

Green Power Smoothie with Spinach and Kale

Ingredients:

- 1 cup fresh spinach leaves
- 1/2 cup kale, stems removed
- 1/2 banana
- 1/2 green apple, chopped
- 1/2 cucumber, peeled and sliced
- 1 cup almond milk
- Ice cubes (optional)

Instructions:

1. Place all ingredients in a blender.

2. Blend until smooth.

3. Pour into a glass and enjoy!

Nutrition Information:

- Calories: 120
- Protein: 4g
- Carbohydrates: 20g
- Fat: 3g
- Fiber: 5g
- Sugar: 10g
- Portion Size: 1 serving

Berry Blast Smoothie with Greek Yogurt

Ingredients:

- 1/2 cup mixed berries (strawberries, blueberries, raspberries)
- 1/2 cup Greek yogurt
- 1/2 banana
- 1 tablespoon chia seeds
- 1 cup water or coconut water

- Ice cubes (optional)

Instructions:

1. Combine all ingredients in a blender.

2. Blend until smooth.

3. Pour into a glass and savor the berry goodness!

Nutrition Information:

- Calories: 150

- Protein: 8g

- Carbohydrates: 25g

- Fat: 4g

- Fiber: 7g

- Sugar: 12g

- Portion Size: 1 serving

Tropical Paradise Smoothie with Coconut Water

Ingredients:

- 1/2 cup pineapple chunks

- 1/2 cup mango chunks

- 1/2 banana
- 1/2 cup coconut water
- 1 tablespoon flaxseeds
- Ice cubes (optional)

Instructions:

1. Put all ingredients in a blender.
2. Blend until smooth.
3. Pour into a glass and transport yourself to a tropical paradise!

Nutrition Information:

- Calories: 140
- Protein: 5g
- Carbohydrates: 30g
- Fat: 3g
- Fiber: 6g
- Sugar: 15g
- Portion Size: 1 serving

Avocado and Mango Smoothie

Ingredients:

- 1/2 ripe avocado
- 1/2 cup mango chunks
- 1/2 cup spinach leaves
- 1/2 cup almond milk
- 1 tablespoon honey
- Ice cubes (optional)

Instructions:

1. Combine all ingredients in a blender.
2. Blend until creamy and smooth.
3. Pour into a glass and relish the rich blend of avocado and mango!

Nutrition Information:

- Calories: 180
- Protein: 5g
- Carbohydrates: 22g
- Fat: 10g
- Fiber: 7g
- Sugar: 12g

- Portion Size: 1 serving

Almond Butter and Banana Protein Smoothie

Ingredients:

- 1 banana
- 2 tablespoons almond butter
- 1/2 cup Greek yogurt
- 1 scoop protein powder
- 1 cup almond milk
- Ice cubes (optional)

Instructions:

1. Place all ingredients in a blender.
2. Blend until smooth and creamy.
3. Pour into a glass and enjoy a protein-packed treat!

Nutrition Information:

- Calories: 250
- Protein: 20g
- Carbohydrates: 25g

- Fat: 10g

- Fiber: 5g

- Sugar: 14g

- Portion Size: 1 serving

Cucumber and Mint Refreshing Smoothie

Ingredients:

- 1/2 cucumber, peeled and sliced

- 1/2 cup fresh mint leaves

- 1/2 green apple, chopped

- 1/2 lime, juiced

- 1 cup coconut water

- Ice cubes (optional)

Instructions:

1. Combine all ingredients in a blender.

2. Blend until the mixture is smooth.

3. Pour into a glass and experience a refreshing cucumber and mint delight!

Nutrition Information:

- Calories: 80
- Protein: 2g
- Carbohydrates: 18g
- Fat: 1g
- Fiber: 4g
- Sugar: 10g
- Portion Size: 1 serving

Chocolate Peanut Butter Protein Smoothie

Ingredients:

- 1 scoop chocolate protein powder
- 2 tablespoons peanut butter
- 1 banana
- 1 cup unsweetened almond milk
- Ice cubes (optional)

Instructions:

1. Add all ingredients to a blender.
2. Blend until the mixture is smooth.

3. Pour into a glass and indulge in the delicious blend
    of chocolate and peanut butter!

Nutrition Information:

- Calories: 280
- Protein: 25g
- Carbohydrates: 20g
- Fat: 12g
- Fiber: 5g
- Sugar: 8g
- Portion Size: 1 serving

Pineapple and Ginger Immunity Booster

Ingredients:

- 1/2 cup pineapple chunks
- 1/2 inch fresh ginger, peeled
- 1/2 cup orange juice
- 1/2 cup Greek yogurt
- 1 tablespoon honey
- Ice cubes (optional)

Instructions:

1. Place all ingredients in a blender.

2. Blend until the mixture is smooth.

3. Pour into a glass and enjoy this refreshing immunity-boosting smoothie!

Nutrition Information:

- Calories: 150

- Protein: 6g

- Carbohydrates: 32g

- Fat: 1g

- Fiber: 3g

- Sugar: 24g

- Portion Size: 1 serving

Blueberry and Oatmeal Breakfast Smoothie

Ingredients:

- 1/2 cup blueberries

- 1/4 cup rolled oats

- 1/2 banana

- 1/2 cup almond milk
- 1 tablespoon flaxseeds
- Ice cubes (optional)

Instructions:

1. Combine all ingredients in a blender.
2. Blend until the mixture is smooth.
3. Pour into a glass and start your day with this nutritious blueberry and oatmeal delight!

Nutrition Information:

- Calories: 200
- Protein: 6g
- Carbohydrates: 35g
- Fat: 5g
- Fiber: 7g
- Sugar: 12g
- Portion Size: 1 serving

Spinach and Pineapple Detox Smoothie

Ingredients:

- 1 cup fresh spinach leaves
- 1/2 cup pineapple chunks
- 1/2 cucumber, peeled and sliced
- 1/2 lemon, juiced
- 1 cup coconut water
- Ice cubes (optional)

Instructions:

1. Add all ingredients to a blender.
2. Blend until the mixture is smooth.
3. Pour into a glass and enjoy this refreshing detoxifying smoothie!

Nutrition Information:

- Calories: 90
- Protein: 3g
- Carbohydrates: 20g
- Fat: 1g
- Fiber: 5g

- Sugar: 10g
- Portion Size: 1 serving

Watermelon and Basil Hydrating Smoothie

Ingredients:

- 1 cup fresh watermelon chunks
- 1/4 cup fresh basil leaves
- 1/2 cup coconut water
- 1/2 lime, juiced
- 1 tablespoon chia seeds
- Ice cubes (optional)

Instructions:

1. Place all ingredients in a blender.
2. Blend until the mixture is smooth.
3. Pour into a glass and relish this hydrating watermelon and basil blend!

Nutrition Information:

- Calories: 70

- Protein: 2g

- Carbohydrates: 18g

- Fat: 1g

- Fiber: 4g

- Sugar: 12g

- Portion Size: 1 serving

Papaya and Lime Smoothie

Ingredients:

- 1/2 cup papaya chunks

- 1/2 banana

- 1/2 cup plain Greek yogurt

- 1/2 lime, juiced

- 1 tablespoon honey

- Ice cubes (optional)

Instructions:

1. Combine all ingredients in a blender.

2. Blend until the mixture is smooth.

3. Pour into a glass and enjoy the tropical flavors of papaya and lime!

Nutrition Information:

- Calories: 120
- Protein: 6g
- Carbohydrates: 25g
- Fat: 2g
- Fiber: 5g
- Sugar: 16g
- Portion Size: 1 serving

Peach and Almond Milk Smoothie

Ingredients:

- 1/2 cup sliced peaches (fresh or frozen)
- 1/2 banana
- 1/2 cup almond milk
- 1 tablespoon almond butter
- 1 teaspoon honey
- Ice cubes (optional)

Instructions:

1. Add all ingredients to a blender.
2. Blend until the mixture is smooth.

3. Pour into a glass and savor the delightful combination of peach and almond milk!

Nutrition Information:

- Calories: 160
- Protein: 5g
- Carbohydrates: 22g
- Fat: 7g
- Fiber: 4g
- Sugar: 14g
- Portion Size: 1 serving

Kiwi and Kale Green Smoothie

Ingredients:

- 1 kiwi, peeled and sliced
- 1/2 cup kale, stems removed
- 1/2 banana
- 1/2 cup pineapple chunks
- 1/2 cup coconut water
- Ice cubes (optional)

Instructions:

1. Place all ingredients in a blender.

2. Blend until the mixture is smooth.

3. Pour into a glass and enjoy the vibrant green goodness of this kiwi and kale smoothie!

Nutrition Information:

- Calories: 110
- Protein: 4g
- Carbohydrates: 25g
- Fat: 2g
- Fiber: 6g
- Sugar: 15g
- Portion Size: 1 serving

Raspberry Coconut Water Electrolyte Smoothie

Ingredients:

- 1/2 cup raspberries
- 1/2 cup coconut water
- 1/2 cup Greek yogurt

- 1 tablespoon chia seeds

- 1 teaspoon honey

- Ice cubes (optional)

Instructions:

1. Combine all ingredients in a blender.

2. Blend until the mixture is smooth.

3. Pour into a glass and enjoy this hydrating raspberry and coconut water electrolyte boost!

Nutrition Information:

- Calories: 120

- Protein: 6g

- Carbohydrates: 20g

- Fat: 3g

- Fiber: 7g

- Sugar: 12g

- Portion Size: 1 serving

CONCLUSION

Throughout the book, we've explored the intricacies of type 2 diabetes and demonstrated how a well-balanced and carefully curated diet can be a powerful tool in the management of blood sugar levels. The 30-day meal plan offers a structured approach to adopting healthier eating habits, encouraging consistency and making the transition to a diabetic-friendly diet seamless.

From energizing breakfasts to satisfying lunches and dinners, our recipes prioritize flavor without compromising on nutritional value. Each dish is thoughtfully crafted to provide a rich tapestry of tastes, textures, and aromas. We've taken care to ensure variety, avoiding repetition to keep every meal exciting and enjoyable.

The inclusion of snacks, appetizers, desserts, and smoothies further reinforces the notion that living with type 2 diabetes does not mean sacrificing the joy of eating. These recipes are a celebration of wholesome ingredients, clever combinations, and culinary creativity, proving that a diabetic diet can be both nourishing and indulgent.

As we conclude this culinary journey, it's our hope that this cookbook becomes a trusted companion in your kitchen, inspiring confidence and promoting a positive relationship with food. Remember, managing type 2 diabetes is not just about restriction; it's about making informed choices that contribute to a vibrant and healthy life.

May this book be a source of inspiration, motivation, and, above all, a testament to the fact that delicious, diabetes-friendly meals are within reach. Cheers to your health, happiness, and the joy of savoring every bite on this flavorful journey towards a balanced and fulfilling life with type 2 diabetes.